THE PROSTATE
and
KEY HEALTH ISSUES
for Older Men

SHAUN DOWLING

authorHOUSE®

AuthorHouse™ UK
1663 Liberty Drive
Bloomington, IN 47403 USA
www.authorhouse.co.uk
Phone: 0800 047 8203 (Domestic TFN)
*   +44 1908 723714 (International)*

Published by AuthorHouse 11/05/2019

ISBN: 978-1-7283-9044-4 (sc)
ISBN: 978-1-7283-9045-1 (hc)
ISBN: 978-1-7283-9043-7 (e)

Library of Congress Control Number: 2019910935

Print information available on the last page.

Any people depicted in stock imagery provided by Getty Images are models, and such images are being used for illustrative purposes only.
Certain stock imagery © Getty Images.

This book is printed on acid-free paper.

Contents

Introduction

The main aim of this book is to raise awareness of certain health disorders, so that older men live their later years in good health. It is not necessarily about living longer, although that would be an additional benefit.

The book describes the ageing process and assesses the risk of certain disorders which may occur. These include the prostate, cancer, heart disease, strokes, osteoporosis, osteoarthritis, diabetes 2 and Alzheimer's; although diabetes 2 is not specifically related to age, it is increasingly common in older men.

As we shall see throughout the studies, early diagnosis can sometimes be critical, so the recent introduction of DNA sequencing to assess health risks will play an important role in future years.

After covering the main disorders, I have gone on to discuss the impact of lifestyle and diet on our heath and suggested what changes could minimise the risk of these disorders occurring in the first place.

CHAPTER 1

HOW OUR BODY WORKS

For those who have not studied biology and physiology the first chapter might be a bit difficult to grasp at first reading, but it is important to take it all in as many of the disorders covered in later chapters can be traced back to the cellular system described here.

Your physical and mental characteristics are inherited from your parents' genes, half from your father, half from your mother. Genes from your mother and the maternal line can be traced back through your mitochondrial DNA to one woman many thousands of years ago. Sometimes you inherit a susceptibility to certain disorders which may affect you in later life. When you see your doctor, he will probably ask you about your family medical history.

So, where and what are the genes in your body? To find out we have to look into your cells.

Your cellular metabolism

Your body comprises billions of eukaryotic cells (as opposed to bacteria cells, discussed below). The exact number, ranging from five billion to several trillions is still in dispute. But what is not disputed is how complex they are. We have around 200 different types of cells, each with different functions, communicating with one another to make the body work. Every cell is enclosed in a permeable membrane which allows gases and fluids to pass between them. Each cell has a nucleus, containing all our genetic material and also mitochondria encased in cytoplasm, part fluid and part tiny organs.

An Eukaryotic Cell

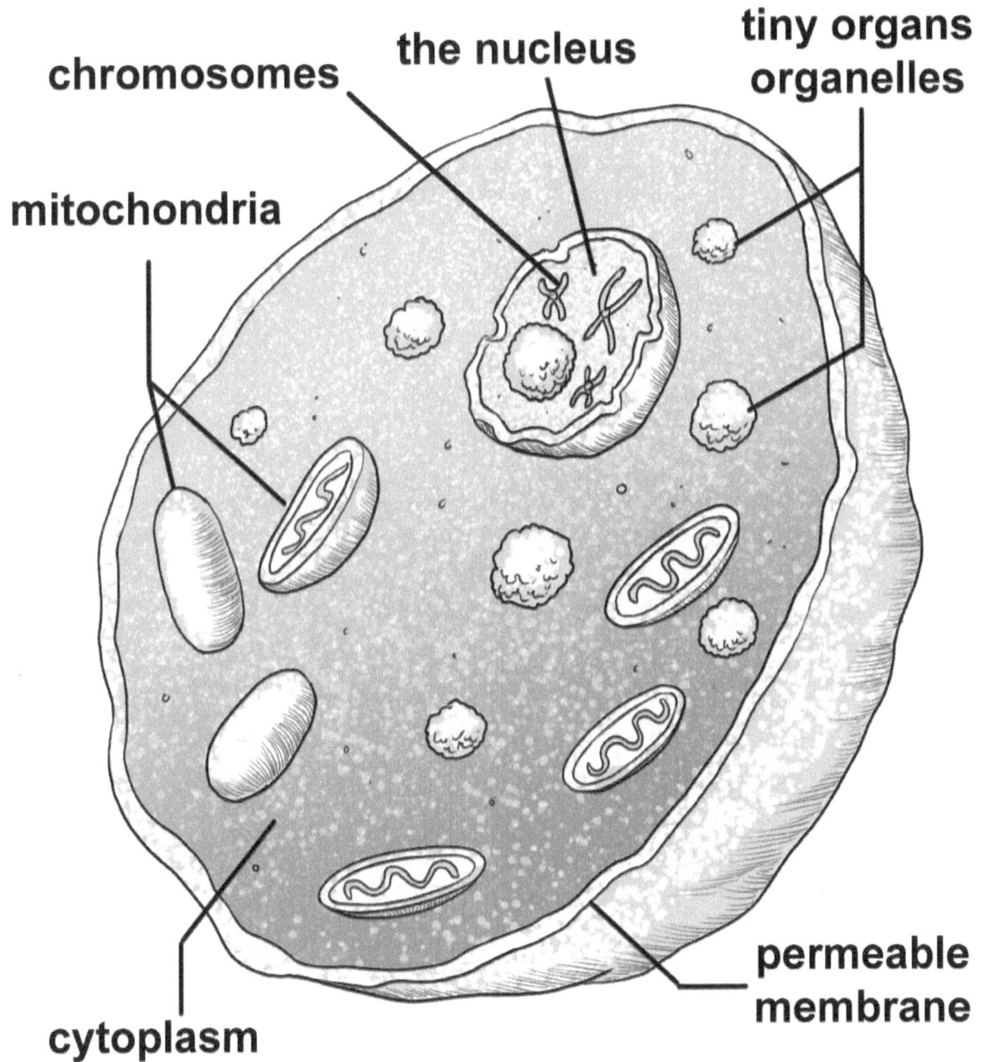

The Genes

Inside the nucleus of each cell there are about 20,000 pairs of genes, which control the growth, functions and repairs of the cell. The genes are arranged in 22 pairs of chromosomes, one each from the father, one from the mother, plus two sex chromosomes.

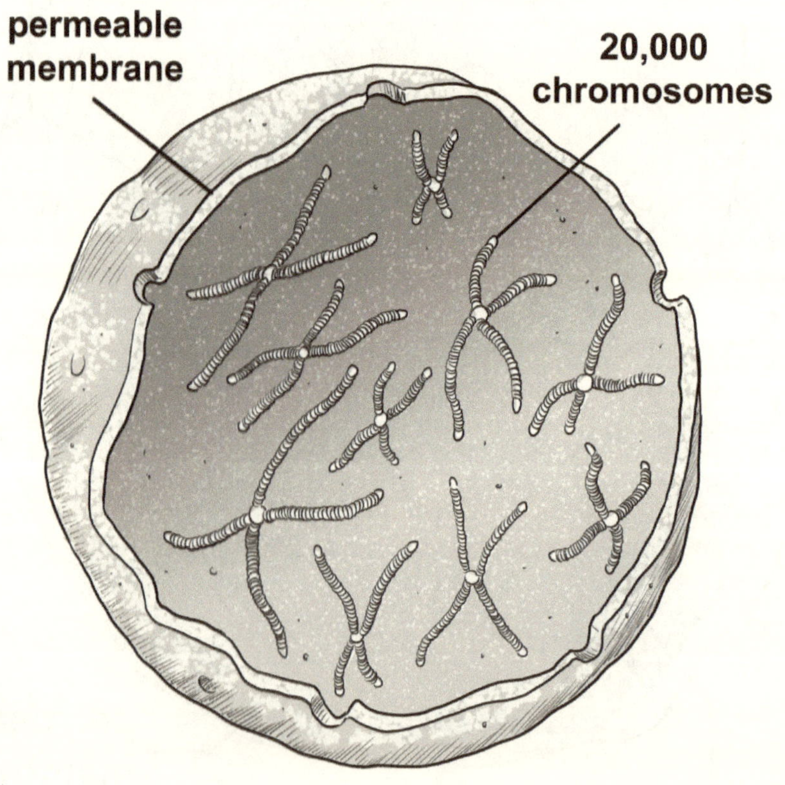

Each chromosome is made up of DNA molecules, shaped like a very long twisted spiral ladder, called a double helix, with rungs of molecules along two strands providing instructions to make proteins and other molecules. These control all our cellular processes. The two strands of the helix are open-ended with protective tips (telomeres) at each end.

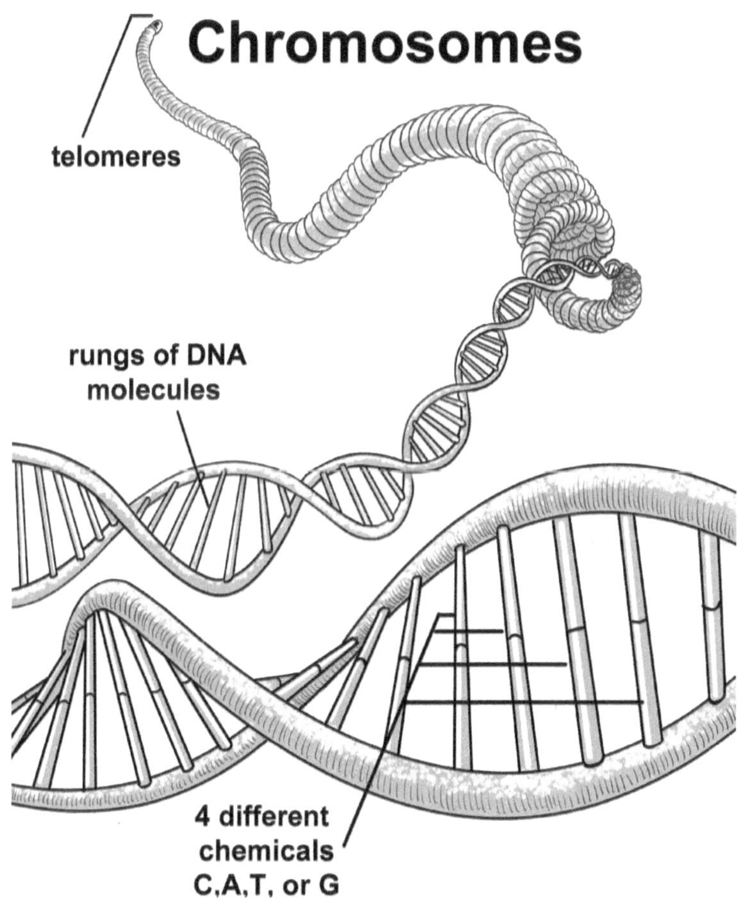

These DNA instructions along the strands of the helix take the form of millions of nucleotides, of which there are only four different chemicals, abbreviated to the letters C, A, T or G. These line up in clusters of three, so there are only 64 possible letter combinations. Snippets of these DNA strands can be read to determine their sequence, and this sequence can now be used for medical diagnosis, forensic identification and paternity testing. So, by taking samples of cells from blood or saliva, you can now get your whole DNA tested to identify any risk of certain diseases as you get older.

Cell Division

The cells are constantly dividing and multiplying, with millions of new cells being produced every minute, although some cells, like skeletal cells, do not divide. Cells can divide up to fifty times, but slow down as we get older and eventually get worn out. When the cells get worn out they are signalled to commit suicide, which is called apoptosis, a vital cellular function as we shall see later. Once they die, the cells disintegrate and the remains are mopped up by neighbouring cells. Each time the cells divide, the telomeres get shorter, which is an indication, but not a cause of ageing. However, cancer cells are able to divide and multiply without being signalled to do so, and their telomeres do not shorten.

In the process of dividing, the chromosomes pair up and the DNA letters get duplicated by an enzyme called polymerase. But that does not always happen correctly, and mistakes are made. When mistakes are made, DNA mutations occur, which, as we see later, can lead to cancer and other medical conditions.

A Mitocondrion

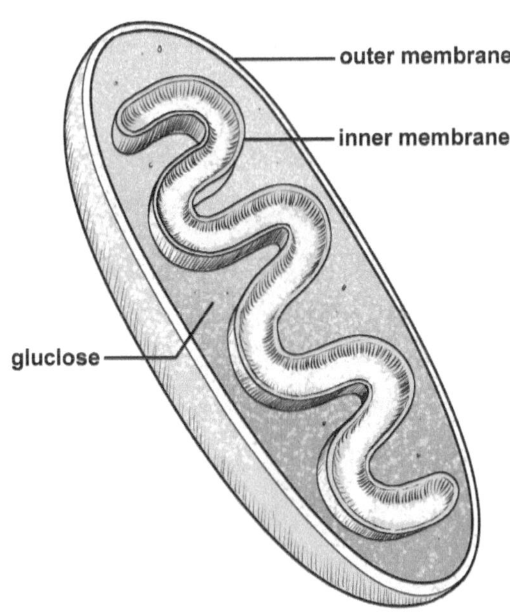

Mitochondria

All this constant cellular activity requires energy, and this is where mitochondria come in. There are hundreds or thousands of mitochondria inside each cell, the number dependent on what the cell needs to do. A single mitochondrion has an outer and convoluted inner membrane where all the energy is produced from the nutrients in our diet. The nutrients needed for energy in our diet are glucose, broken down from carbohydrate, and fat, converted into glycerol and fatty acid. Glucose is transported from our blood stream into our mitochondria by a hormone called insulin, secreted from the beta cells in our pancreas. In a complicated chemical process, called glycolysis, one molecule of glucose, plus oxygen from our respiratory system and blood stream produces up to 38 molecules of ATP (adenosine triphosphate).

In a slightly different process, fatty acid is metabolised to produce ATP, which it does more productively than glucose, producing up to 129 molecules of ATP for one molecule of fatty acid. However, whereas glucose can get straight into the mitochondria to start the energy process, fatty acid needs a transporter called L-carnitine, to pass it through the outer mitochondrial membrane.

ATP

ATP is the body's key and only energy molecule which, in aerobic respiration, causes our muscles to move. ATP can also be produced without oxygen in a slightly different chemical process, called anaerobic respiration but it is far less efficient and can only be sustained for short periods, as many athletes, when short of breath, can testify. ATP cannot be stored, and its turnover is very rapid, as each ATP molecule survives for only seconds before it is replicated.

The Electronic Chain

Conversion of glucose or fatty acid into ATP and then into energy is where another problem arises. The whole process uses a complex 5-stage Electronic Transport Chain (ETC). We don't need to go into detail how ETC works, but suffice to say, when our demands for energy are high the electrons flow down the chain quickly, but when we need little energy the electrons can back up, some escape from the chain and form superoxide free radicals. A chain reaction then occurs in which a free radical steals an electron from another molecule, and that steals an electron from another molecule, and so on. Fortunately, our bodies also produce antioxidant molecules, which give up electrons to free radicals without themselves being destabilised. For our health, the idea is to keep a balance between free radicals and antioxidants. When there are more free radicals than antioxidants our cells suffer oxidative stress, leading to mutations to our DNA, which other protein molecules may be unable to repair.

When we look at our varying energy needs, from lying in bed to intensive sports, we little realise that our need for ATP is continuous, as our organs are working hard for 24 hours a day. Even we we are asleep, the brain is using up 20% of our energy, whilst our heart muscles are operating at the same level as they do for most of the day. But if we consume more nutrients than we need at the time, not only does the ETC get blocked, with free radicals escaping, but the excess glucose gets stored in the liver in the form of glycogen. If the glycogen is not used up by more activity, it builds up as body fat. However, in its defence, body fat can provide convenient storage as it can be reconverted into glucose for use at a later date.

Muscle Movement

To complete the process from intake of nutrients into physical energy, we should take a brief look at the process from ATP to muscle movement. We have two types of muscles, skeletal, which move our bones and joints around and smooth muscles which control our organs and blood circulatory system. Skeletal muscles take the form of bundles of thin fibres. Inside these fibres are tiny strands of protein filaments. On command from neurotransmitters in the brain, protein filaments slide past one another, the muscle contracts and movement occurs. Muscles can only contract and relax. In most cases the muscles operate in pairs, one contracting, the other relaxing.

Cholesterol

No study of our cellular metabolism would be complete without looking at how the cell membranes are built up, kept flexible and permeable. The lipid molecule which does this is called cholesterol, circulating in the blood stream. Cholesterol has other functions than building cell membranes. It is involved in cell signalling, fighting inflammation, forming synapses in the brain, neutralising free radicals and synthesising Vitamin D and many hormones.

As cholesterol is insoluble, it has to be transported within protein particles called lipoproteins. Cholesterol is mostly synthesised in the body, but can also be absorbed from eating animal based foods, like meat, fish, cheese and eggs. 80% of cholesterol is produced in and later secreted from the liver. There are two main types of cholesterol, LDL (low density lipoprotein) and HDL (high density lipoprotein), but also VLDL (very low-density lipoprotein), all of which add up to Total Cholesterol.

Cholesterol levels rise and fall during the day, and between summer and winter. The normal level for total cholesterol is measured at about 5.2 mmol/L. High levels are 6.2 mmol/L and above. LDL cholesterol is known to be part of the plaques which build up on the walls of the arteries, leading to atherosclerosis, but on the positive side it helps to repair inflammatory damage to the artery walls and its proponents say that it serves as a healing agent. HDL in particular is known to reduce atherosclerosis. The debate about cholesterol continues, but I think the general consensus today is that LDL is the 'bad' cholesterol and HDL the 'good' cholesterol. Certain doctors get worried if total cholesterol goes over 7 mmol/L or HDL falls below 1.3 mmol/L and they may prescribe regular aspirin or statins.

(Oddly enough, the World Health Organisation has reported that countries with the highest levels of cholesterol have the lowest death rates from heart disease, whilst those with the lowest levels have the highest death rates.)

Bacteria Cells

So far in this chapter we have described eukaryotic cells but have not mentioned bacteria cells, their forerunners, which were originally involved in energy production before mitochondria evolved. Bacteria cells do not contain a nucleus, but do contain a cell wall, a cell membrane, cytoplasm and circular, but not open ended DNA. There are about a thousand different types of bacteria cells, mainly in our gut and on our skin, of which about forty are most prominent.

Bacteria play an important role in our digestive system, synthesising vitamins, fermenting dietary fibre and regulating our immune system, but they can also cause bacterial infections. Certain drugs, or overuse of drugs, can damage our gut bacteria so they become antibiotic resistant. It is important to keep our gut bacteria, or gut flora, in good condition, which we will cover in Chapter 9.

The Ageing Process

What have we learnt so far from our study of the body's metabolism that relates to ageing? From the outside, the changes are obvious. The skin wrinkles, hair falls out, our posture deteriorates and there may be some cognitive impairment.

Inside the body, the tissues stiffen and become less elastic, particularly in the respiratory tract, so our lung capacity decreases. Our blood sugars also rise and this requires more insulin, which can lead to insulin resistance and diabetes. Our cells get worn down and the process of cell division and replication also slows down. The telomeres at the end of our chromosomes get shorter, an indication of ageing, and the process of apoptosis, described above, killing off senescent cells, becomes less efficient. But it is likely that the main cause of ageing is the cumulative damage, or mutations, to our DNA which other protein molecules are unable to repair. To support this theory, studies of centenarians have shown that they retain a significantly higher level of DNA repair proteins than younger people.

This seems a rather dreary list of metabolic changes which occur as we get older but there are some things which we can do to slow this process down, as we shall see in Chapters 9 and 10.

In the meantime the pharmaceutical industry is desperately trying to develop drugs which will slow down the ageing process, although I cannot hazard a guess whether they will be successful.

Interestingly, calorific restriction and periodic fasting is known to prolong the life of most animals, but there is no proof yet that this applies to humans.

C H A P T E R 2

THE PROSTATE

I am very happy to report on the prostate as this subject was not widely discussed in public until 20 or 30 years ago.

As men get older the prostate grows in size and eventually restricts the urethra, the tube leading down from the bladder to the penis which allows you to urinate. The growth is caused by cells in the prostate dividing and replicating, as they do elsewhere in the body. Why they do this is not properly known, but is likely to be related to the change in our sex hormones as we age, since the prostate is involved in the production of sperm in our semen, and it may also be due to the weakening of our muscular tissues. Those who were castrated as children never get an enlarged prostate.

The prostate in young men is about the size of a walnut, but can grow three or four times that size. This not only squeezes the urethra, but causes older men to urinate frequently, perhaps three or four times a night. It can sometimes be painful or difficult to urinate, and usually the bladder cannot be completely emptied. Doctors can tell how large the prostate has become, by putting a finger up the anus, which is closely aligned to the prostate.

In medical terms an enlarged prostate is called Benign Prostate Hyperplasia (BPH) but unfortunately the prostate is not always benign and cancer may be present, particularly in some ethnic groups. It has been said that cancer is present to some degree in most older men and if they live to be 120, they could die if it was not treated. Whether or not your prostate is cancerous can be indicated by an ultrasound or MRI, and can be confirmed by a biopsy. One other indication, which is sadly rather unreliable, is the reading of a PSA (prostate specific antigen) test. The PSA level, per se, is less indicative of cancer than the annual increase. If, say, it rises by 1 point from 6 to 7, it should be investigated.

If you have non-cancerous enlargement of the prostate (BPH) what are the options? Firstly, whether to have treatment or not. You can carry on with the inconvenience and discomfort, which may not get any worse, or go for some treatment. If you decide to do nothing for the moment, watch out for a urine infection or problems with the kidneys or bladder. Your doctor may advise you to take tablets, like alpha blocker inhibitors, although these take some time to take effect. If you decide for surgery, a urologist will first want to have a look at both the prostate and the bladder. This can be done with a flexible cystoscopy in which a miniature telescope can be inserted through the urethra and pictures can be taken of the prostate and the bladder.

If you just have BPH you don't need to take the prostate out. There are various other procedures, as follows:

TURP: transurethral resection of the prostate
PVP: photoselective vapourisation of the prostate
HOLEP: Holmium laser enucleation of the prostate
PAE: prostate artery embolisation of the prostate

The traditional TURP operation involves surgical removal of the core of the prostate, and probably involves 2 or 3 days in hospital. This treatment is often referred to as 'the gold standard.' Both PVP and HOLEP use laser vaporisation, which is less intrusive and may only involve an overnight stay in hospital. After the operation, patients are not usually allowed home until the urethra is working properly. In some cases, the blood or debris from the operation blocks the urethra, the patient cannot pass water and so a catheter with a tap may need to be inserted for a few days until the urethra is completely clear. PAE, using a microsphere to block artery access to the prostate is the least invasive, but a urologist should advise what treatment is suitable.

If you have prostate cancer, the symptoms are the same as for BPH, except of course it is not benign. The cancer may have been discovered after having a BPH operation when the core of the prostate is examined by a pathologist, or it could have been found out from scans or a biopsy. The severity of prostate cancer is graded according to a Gleeson scoring system from 0 to 10 when a pathologist looks at two predominant patterns in the tissues and adds them together. A score of 5 and over is classed as aggressive for which treatment is recommended. For those with a score of 1 to 4, it is possible to continue with active monitoring, in particular checking that the PSA is not rising and also having regular scans.

If treatment is required, the first call is to have radiotherapy in which the cancer cells are killed, but the disadvantage is that it will kill off normal cells as well. Radiotherapy can be undertaken with high energy X-rays or implanting radioactive seeds in the prostate. In either case, patients will feel more fatigued and many have some discomfort passing urine. There is also a risk of weight gain and reduced sexual potency.

A further alternative is to have hormone therapy in which a cancer tumour is deprived of testosterone and cancer cells die off. Some patients may have this before or after radiotherapy. This treatment does cause hot flushes, weight gain and reduced sexual potency. Hormone therapy could be continued for years but may not completely eradicate the cancer.

One further option is total removal of the prostate, a prostatectomy, which affects sexual potency and may also lead to incontinence. And finally, for advanced cancer, the testicles can be removed, which rapidly reduces the testosterone. In all cases of cancer, observation and scans are needed to see that the cancer has not metastasised to any other part of the body.

CHAPTER 3

HEART DISORDERS

First, let us take a look at how the heart works, then go on to see what can go wrong and how to deal with it.

The heart is a fist sized pump, only weighing about 1 lb, which circulates the blood round the body in about one minute at rest. The circulation speeds up as we exercise. The heart is centrally situated, not on the left as many believe. The heart is surrounded by a three-layer wall, or membrane, in the middle of which lies the myocardial muscle which drives the pump. This muscle is the key to normal living, and any damage or infection can be dangerous.

The heart has four chambers, two upper atria and two lower ventricles, operating two different circuits. In one circuit the left ventricle pumps oxygenated blood through the aorta into the arteries and capillaries, giving up oxygen and nutrients, whilst the right atrium collects deoxygenated blood and carbon dioxide from the veins. In the second circuit, the right ventricle pumps blood to and from the lungs to collect oxygen and wash out carbon dioxide. The capillaries are the key component in this exchange system. Being porous, they can exchange oxygen, carbon dioxide, glucose, amino acids and hormones.

The pump operates at about 70 beats per minute at rest, regulated by electrical impulses from the sinoatrial node (the pacemaker), but it takes a whole minute for all the blood to be circulated. The blood itself consists of plasma, corpuscles and minute platelets. The plasma is mainly water with nutrients dissolved in it it. The corpuscles are red and white cells, the red mainly used for transport of oxygen to the cells, the white used for fighting infections, including cancer. All the arteries, veins and capillaries are coated with a lining consisting of a layer of cells called the endothelium. If any blood vessels are damaged the platelets come together to seal the linings.

There are a number of heart disorders which have similar symptoms and similar causes. These symptoms can include raised or irregular heart beat, headaches, dizziness, sweating, palpitations, blurred vision, shortness of breath, chest pain and even swollen feet and ankles, although no disorder creates all of these symptoms. The causes can be congenital but are mainly related to age, lifestyle, diet and stress.

As we age, our tissues stiffen, our arteries harden and airways in the respiratory system become less elastic, leading to a reduction in lung capacity; our maximum heart rate declines and our muscles weaken, particularly our cardiac muscles. As our lung capacity decreases, we become more susceptible to bronchitis, pneumonia, emphysema and other pulmonary disorders.

Most of us know about our heart rate from feeling our pulse. Our blood pressure is usually measured in the doctor's surgery by a sphygmomanometer. The highest measure (systolic pressure) is about 120 mmHg or above when the heart muscles contract, and the lowest (diastolic pressure) is about 80 mmHg or above when the heart muscles relax. In a young man, you would expect a blood pressure reading of around 120/80 at rest. This creeps up as we age and the systolic pressure is sometimes estimated at 220 mmHg minus our age. So, for an 80-year old, it might be 140/90.

Hypertension

When we come to heart disorders, most of them affect, rather than are caused by failure of the heart mechanism described above and could equally be called 'circulatory disorders'. First and foremost is hypertension, or high blood pressure. For some it could be hereditary, but for most of us it is caused by age, weight, lifestyle and stress. Whilst our arteries become more rigid as we age, the greatest damage arises from narrowing of the arteries, restricting blood flow to the heart and causing damage to the heart muscles. Physical symptoms of hypertension may include headaches, dizziness and blurred vision, or you may not notice anything until you are checked by a doctor. Mild hypertension is generally reversible by stopping smoking, cutting down on alcohol, losing weight and undertaking sufficient exercise.

Angina and Atherosclerosis

Hypertension is often a warning sign for more serious heart problems to come. If you get chest pains during light exercise, like climbing stairs or walking up a hill, you probably have Angina. Atherosclerosis, or narrowing or the arteries, is where plaques or clots develop on the endothelium, the lining of the artery walls. These clots are said to be due to an excess of cholesterol in the blood but the clots also consist of other components, including blood plasma, dead cells and insoluble proteins. Whilst blood clotting is important for stopping bleeding and forming a protective seal over injuries, it can be most unhelpful in the arteries where clots occur. If the clot is attached to the artery wall it is called a thrombus, but if it gets detached and moves round the blood vessels it is classed as a more dangerous embolus.

Whilst angina can be treated with drugs, atherosclerosis needs further investigation. You would be likely to have an ECG (electrocardiogram) which traces the electrical activity in your heart, both at rest and during exercise. To find out where the clots are you would need an angiograph procedure in which dye is injected into the arteries and X-rays taken. Once that is done, you might have an angioplasty. This procedure widens the artery, which has narrowed, or become blocked. A balloon catheter is passed through the artery, blown up and a tubular structure called a stent is left in place. Stents are now commonly used, even in mild cases of atherosclerosis. In more serious cases you could need a coronary artery by-pass graft (CABG), when a section of a blood vessel, taken from your chest or legs, is grafted onto your artery where the damage occurred. In extreme cases, the heart itself may be replaced, although it is said there are not enough hearts available for this operation.

Heart Attack

A heart attack (myocardial infarction) occurs when a clot has completely blocked the coronary artery. There is a crushing pain in the chest, shortness of breath, nausea and extreme anxiety. Part of the heart muscle ceases to work as there is no oxygenated blood available. In some cases, the heart actually stops beating and this cannot be sustained for more than a few minutes without resuscitation. Medical attention is needed immediately. Before an ambulance arrives, taking a 300 mg aspirin will help. Usually a patient will recover, but there may be long term damage to the heart muscle. In this case further drugs and anticoagulants are likely to be needed. Medical advice is sure to be given on diet, alcohol, stress and lifestyle.

Other Heart Disorders

Before or after a heart attack you could have a form of heart failure in which the heart pump is not efficient; this leads to poor circulation and accumulated fluid in the lungs known as pulmonary oedema, and may lead to pulmonary disease. Initially, one or other side of the heart may be affected. Another heart disorder is atrial fibrillation, in which the heart muscle is weakened. In this case both the atria and the ventricles, which are supposed to work together do not operate in a co-ordinated way and the heart beats much more rapidly than normal. This occurs mostly in older people and local surgeries now encourage older people to have an ECG. Sometimes it is the heart valves themselves than cause the problem. The valves may have been damaged by an infection or a previous heart attack, but usually the valves can be repaired or replaced by a mechanical or pig's valve. The severity of a valve defect can be measured by an echocardiogram,using an ultrasound probe on the chest.

Abnormal heart rates are called arrhythmias. Where the heart rate is too high it is called tachycardia; too low, it is called bradycardia. Bradycardia can even exist in athletes during intense training. Any abnormality of this kind will reduce the efficiency of the pumping mechanism. Usually arrhythmias are caused by some form of heart disease, atrial fibrillation, valve disorders or synoatrial node malfunction, which can cause an irregular pulse.

There are a host of less common, but not inconsequential heart disorders affecting the heart, the valves and the vascular system, where other parts of the body are affected. In advanced diabetes, for example, the legs can be seriously affected. In deep vein thrombosis (DVT) an embolus, or detached clot, can travel to, and block the veins in the legs. This is caused by long periods of immobility, say on a long flight or car journey, where the legs aren't moved around.

All heart disorders require treatment, but the most important step is to recognise the problem. Sometimes people do nothing until it gets serious, then go and see a doctor. If you recognise a health issue, you are half way to solving it.From then on it's medication and changes in lifestyle.

C HAPTER 4

STROKES

A stroke, or cardiovascular accident can either be caused by a blockage of the blood supply to the brain, called an ischaemic stroke (or transient ischaemic attack) or else by a haemorrhage when a blood vessel in the brain leaks or bursts. The former is most common, 80%, the latter 20%. Sometimes the blockage occurs inside the brain; at other times a embolus, or clot, travels from another part of the body. In either case, part of the brain stops working and urgent attention is needed. Men are more liable to strokes than women, particularly as they get older. The risk of a stroke almost doubles every decade for men over 65.

There are even more causes for a stroke than a heart attack. These include high blood pressure, high cholesterol, smoking, diabetes 2, obesity, lack of exercise, stress, atrial fibrillation, infection, illicit drugs, sickle cell disease and carotid stenosis (narrowing of the carotid artery). Symptoms of an ischaemic stroke are facial weakness, slow speech, paralysis of one side of the body, loss of balance, blurred vision, or, worst of all, loss of consciousness. The main symptom for a haemorrhagic stroke is a severe headache, sometimes followed by vomiting and could lead to a coma. A stroke will affect particular parts of the brain, which create different symptoms – a useful indicator for diagnosis. If the left side of the brain is damaged, the right side of the body will be affected, and vice versa.

The type of stroke will determine the treatment given. Brain imaging will be needed by an MRI or CT scan and a cerebral angiogram may be performed with injected dye to identify the location of the clot. A clot may be removed using a special catheter inserted into the blood vessels in the groin, then threaded through the body into the brain (a thrombectomy) or by intravenous treatment to dissolve the clot. In some cases, a craniotomy could be performed, opening up the skull to relieve pressure and remove accumulated blood. One difference between strokes and heart attacks is that strokes have a nasty habit of repeating, so the type of treatment and the use of drugs or coagulants has to be carefully monitored.

Patients with strokes can usually leave hospital quite quickly, but full rehabilitation often takes time. There may still be problems of movement, swallowing, incontinence, tiredness, depression and poor memory, requiring medical attention. Recommendations for changing lifestyle given by the doctors will be much the same as for patients with heart disorders. Some suggestions are shown in Chapters 9 and 10.

Chapter 5

OSTEOARTHRITIS AND OSTEOPOROSIS

<u>Osteoarthritis</u>

Osteoarthritis is inflammation of the synovial joints in the bones, affecting the surrounding tissue, muscles and cartilage. The onset of osteoarthritis is usually gradual and progressive. The joints most at risk are the hands, wrists, knees, hips and back. Each joint is encased in a synovium, lubricated by synovial fluid. As the disorder progresses, the cartilage gets thinner and the bones on either side get thicker. The joints do not move as smoothly as they should which puts pressure on the surrounding tendons and ligaments connected to the bones.

Older women are twice as likely to develop osteoarthritis as older men, particularly in their hands and knees. This may be due to the fall in their oestrogen levels. As we age, our

33

fitness declines, the muscles get weaker and the body is less able to repair damage to the cartilage. Those with a family history of osteoarthritis are more likely to suffer from this disorder. Other causes are repeated minor injuries, rupture of the crucial ligament and excessive weight. Many athletes suffer from osteoarthritis on their hips and knees after a long period in contact sports. Those who are overweight also put more pressure on their joints and muscles. It is also thought that a deficiency in calcium and Vitamins C, D and E, may be a contributory cause of osteoarthritis.

The symptoms of osteoarthritis are pain, swelling, cracking joints and tenderness to touch. If you see your doctor, he will probably look into your medical and family history, check your bone alignment, give you a blood test and send you for an MRI scan or X-ray. Apart from giving you tablets or pain killers, there is not much else he can do, but advise you to manage the disorder yourself. This means taking gentle exercise and keeping your weight down. Swimming is the best exercise as it reduces the load on your body, but yoga and T'ai Chi are also recommended. You might also look at vitamin supplements, or tablets of glucosamine and chondroitin, which is alleged to hydrate the cartilage and improve joint flexibility.

Osteoarthritis should not be confused with rheumatoid arthritis, which has some of the same symptoms. Rheumatoid arthritis is an autoimmune disorder in which antibodies attack the synovial membrane, causing damage to the cartilage and tendons. This too runs in some families and is about three times more common in women than men. The diagnosis would be similar to that for osteoporosis, location of swelling, blood test and X-rays. Treatment would include drugs, physiotherapy and recommendation for gentle exercise.

Osteoporosis

Osteoporosis is a disorder affecting loss of bone density. The bones get thinner and more fragile, with a higher risk of fracture, particularly in the wrists, hips or spine. The bone structure is made of about 85% collagen and 15% other proteins. Biologically, bones are more active than we might imagine. Bones both lose and gain mass throughout our lifetime, so there is actually a bone turnover. The turnover can be measured in blood and urine tests. The thickness of the bone structure is mainly due to genetic factors but diet, exercise and health issues can play a part. Bone mass is at its highest around the age of 30. From middle age onwards, you lose up to 1% a year of your bone mass, so your skeleton could be nearly a third lighter at 70 than at 40!

The two main cells involved in building new bone are osteoblasts and osteocytes. If there is bone loss, collagen molecules are released and can be measured in blood and urine. A gain in bone mass is due to a process involving hormones, oestrogen, steroids and Vitamin D, the vitamin which controls the absorption of calcium and phosphate. Bone turnover is not yet fully understood but is known to be affected by our nutritional intake.

The need for a diagnosis may follow a fall, a fracture or localised pain. A diagnosis will probably involve blood tests, X-rays, a scan by a DXA machine and possibly a bone biopsy. Prevention of osteoporosis can be helped by a good diet, including adequate calcium and Vitamin D intake, also by walking and weight bearing exercise. Conversely, smoking and excess alcohol have a damaging effect. Treatment may also require medication, physiotherapy, hydrotherapy and relaxation therapies.

CHAPTER 6

DIABETES

The exact cause of Diabetes 2 is not known, but it is characterised by high blood sugar, common in those who are overweight, particularly those over 40. It also runs in families and ethnic groups. Diabetes 1 has some of the same symptoms as Diabetes 2, but is less common, more serious and mainly affects younger people. Here we shall only deal with Diabetes 2.

Our blood sugar is controlled by the hormone insulin, secreted from beta cells in the pancreas. Blood sugar is created mainly from glucose, converted from carbohydrate in our diet, then used for energy in the metabolic process described in Chapter 1. Excess glucose is stored in our liver as glycogen. The beta cells are supposed to monitor the whole metabolic process and secrete insulin according to need, but sometimes it does not work properly and there is a slow build up of blood sugar, which leads to insulin resistance. Likewise, if the pancreas is damaged, infected, diseased or overloaded with drugs or alcohol, the beta cells will not operate efficiently.

The normal level of blood sugar is about 4 to 5 mmol/L. It usually rises 1 to 2 hours after a meal, then falls as physical activity and body maintenance burns up the fuel. As we get older, and if we eat more food than we need, we put on more weight, our insulin hormone gets less efficient, the mitochondrial membranes get blocked up and if our blood sugar rises over 12 mmol/L, the kidneys secrete the excess glucose from our blood into our urine.

Insulin resistance not only leads to Diabetes 2, but also to hypertension, the starting point for heart disease. It also weakens the immune system and lowers HDL, the 'good' cholesterol. Diabetes 2 often creeps up slowly and it is not always picked up until a blood test or urine test is given. Meanwhile there may be symptoms of excessive thirst, frequent passing of urine, urinary or skin infections and general fatigue.

According to the World Health Organisation the incidence of Diabetes quadrupled between 1980 and 2018, rather hard to believe, but probably partly attributable to better diagnosis and reporting. In the UK it is forecast to use up 17% of the NHS budget by 2035. It is most unlikely that this increase is due to family predisposition to Diabetes, more likely to the increase in obesity which accounts for 80% to 85% of cases. In the USA, for example, it is said 60% of Americans are overweight, whilst the increase in the UK has also been noticeable. A BMI rating of 25-30 (see page 60) is regarded as overweight, over 30 it is regarded as obese, and over 35 the risk of Diabetes is one hundred times greater than normal. (The BMI Index is set out on page 75). The whole issue of weight and obesity is covered fully in Chapter 9. There we look at our basal metabolic rate and certain genetic risk factors inherited from our parents.

Treatment of Diabetes 2 means getting the blood sugar level down to normal levels, boosting the hormone insulin, eating less, increasing physical activity, avoiding recreational drugs and excess alcohol, and taking the medications recommended. Some medication can be quite simple, like aspirin and statins, whilst drugs can be given to enhance the secretion of insulin. In either case the blood sugar has to be measured on a regular basis. This can be done by patients doing their own testing, whether finger pricking and checking the blood with a test strip, or using a test strip to place in a stream of urine. There is now a needle like flash monitor available which is a sensor, worn on the upper arm, which can read blood sugar levels.

Whilst Diabetes 2 is not curable, it is quite manageable with a change in lifestyle and medication. The biggest risk is an infection or ulcers, particularly in the limbs, and if not treated can lead to nerve damage, weakened bones, poor circulation and vascular disease. In a worst case it could lead to amputations. So those who are seriously overweight should watch out in case any symptoms develop, control their diet and keep their blood pressure down.

CHAPTER 7

CANCER

Cancer is a metabolic disorder, starting in the mitochondria, whereby cell growth becomes uncontrolled and may metastasise to other parts of the body. Only one cell, and we have millions of them, is enough to start the process. There are over a hundred types of cancer; the main cancers for men in the UK being prostate, lung, colorectal, skin, stomach, melanoma and pancreas.

Cancer is the main cause of mortality, although this is now falling by 1% per year. Survival for men is 75% for prostate, 50% for colon but only 6.5% for lung cancer. Over the age of 60, three in one hundred are diagnosed with cancer each year. A change in lifestyle could reduce the risk of cancer. Cancer Research UK estimates that 42% of cancers are potentially preventable. We shall look into this below.

The Nucleus

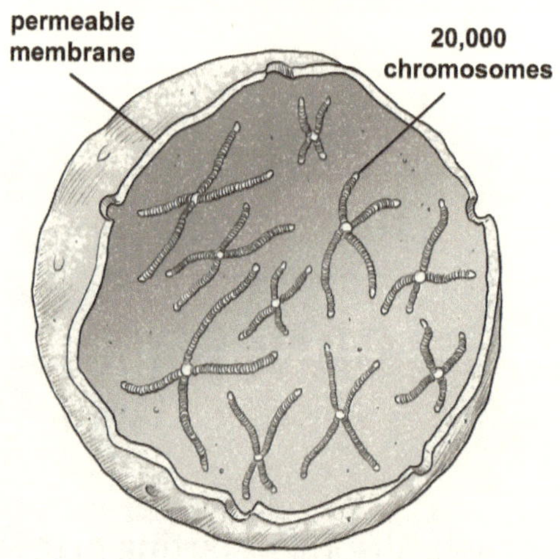

DNA Mutations

The first step in understanding the risks of cancer is to go back to the description of the genes and DNA in Chapter 1. All of our genetic material is contained in the nucleus of our eukaryotic cells. In each cell we have over 20,000 pairs of genes which control cellular growth, division, function and repairs. When the cells divide, the chromosomes pair up and get duplicated, normally with the same code of DNA instructions. This does not always happen correctly and DNA mutations occur. However, this is not the only cause of DNA mutations. Some can be inherited from our parents. Some are caused by free radicals damaging our DNA, which our DNA proteins are unable to repair. Some are damaged by exposure to carcinogens (cancer agents). Carcinogens include tobacco smoke, pollution, UV sunlight, radiation from X-rays, some viruses, excess alcohol and food toxins. Some cells are more exposed to carcinogens than others, particularly those that line our lungs, skin, bowel and stomach. One APOBEC enzyme, which normally protects us from viruses, sometimes attacks the DNA and this also causes mutations.

Mutations can usually be repaired by other DNA protein molecules within the cell. But as mutations accumulate, the cells get worn out and the cell is signalled to self destruct by committing suicide (apoptosis), in which case the remaining cell fragments are mopped up by neighbouring cells. If a cell ignores the signal to die, it can become malignant. Typically, it takes around 8-10 mutations in a cell to become malignant and cancerous, but active screening of cells by the immune system usually induces apoptosis before this level is reached.

<u>Cancer Cells</u>

Cancer cells have certain characteristics. They resist apoptosis. They don't need proper instructions to double or multiply, and they don't need as much oxygen to grow as normal cells. They seek to avoid white blood cells which would normally destroy them and they can sprout capillaries, in a form of angiogenesis, to enable them to pick up nutrients and oxygen, without which they can not grow. These cells may take years to develop into a recognisable tumour; or they could develop quickly. They are not necessarily life threatening, unless they spread. Most cancers occur in the epithelial cells, on the walls of the arteries, and are called carcinomas. They spread from the capillaries, invading nearby tissue and can metastasize through the lymph nodes, the blood stream or other circulating fluids. In cases of metastasis, prostate cancer can spread to the bones; skin cancer can spread to the liver, lungs and brain; lung cancer can spread to the bones, liver, brain and adrenal glands; and bowel cancer can spread to the liver, lungs and abdominal cavity.

Cancer and Age

The reason that older people are more at risk is because they have collected more mutations during their lifetimes, and it is the accumulation of mutations, and declining efficiency of our immune system, that makes us more vulnerable. Hence the total number of cancer cases worldwide grows as our lifespan increases. However, what surprises and heartens me the most about cancer is that all the billions of cells and trillions of DNA in our bodies, which incur mutations every day, do not lead to a much higher incidence of cancer.

Symptoms

The symptoms of cancer may be hard to spot. There may be a lump or mole on the skin, blood in the urine or faeces, persistent heartburn or headache. There may be difficulty in swallowing, unexplained tiredness, loss of appetite or weight loss. Once these symptoms have been reported, cancer can be diagnosed by screening, blood tests, X-rays, MRI and CT scans and a look at family history. If necessary, a biopsy can be undertaken and it is no longer necessary to take a cut of tissue, as a less invasive liquid biopsy can be taken from the blood.

Treatments

Treatments vary considerably according to the age and condition of the patient, but the most common are chemotherapy, radiotherapy, hormonal treatment, interferon drugs or surgery, accompanied by appropriate pain relief. Chemotherapy can be applied by drugs or injection into the veins on a daily, weekly or monthly basis, over a given period of time. Unfortunately, treatments do have side effects like fatigue, weakness, depression and possible hair loss. The main problem is that, however well chemotherapy and radiation are targeted, they kill off normal cells as well as cancer cells. One new form of radiation is proton beam therapy which targets cancer tumours from two angles and does not damage neighbouring cells to the same extent. This is not yet available for all types of cancer, but is likely to become much more commonly used in the future. However, the main issue is whether it cures the cancer and it does not re-occur for another 5 years. In all cases, follow up investigation is necessary and the medical staff may recommend changes in lifestyle.

The Most Common Cancers

The most common cancers are described in more detail below.

Prostate

Described in detail in Chapter 2, prostate is the most common cancer for men, and affects one in eight during their lifetime. Whilst the cause is not entirely clear, its growth and survival probably depend on the hormone, testosterone. It is usually diagnosed when there are signs of an enlarged prostate. The treatments vary from regular observation to a radical prostatectomy, but radiotherapy and hormone therapy are more common treatments.

Skin

The main cause of skin cancer is exposure to the sun or sunbeds, particularly for fair headed children, although it may not be manifested for many years. In the UK the main types are basal cell, squamous cell and malignant carcinoma. Basal cell carcinoma is the most common, characterised by a slow growing ulcer type lesion on the skin which will not heal. A biopsy is relatively simple, and if cancerous will probably be removed by surgery or PDT (photodynamic therapy). The outcome is usually satisfactory, but further observation is needed to see that it does not re-occur on another part of the body.

Squamous carcinoma is more common in older men, characterised by a reddish brown lump on the face or hands, again requiring surgery, even radiotherapy and chemotherapy if it has spread. Malignant melanoma, more common in women, may develop from a small lump or mole which reddens, grows and may bleed. This is the most aggressive of the skin cancers, needing drugs and radiotherapy or chemotherapy. For all types of skin cancer, once treated, stay out of the sun, cover the body and wear a hat.

<u>Lymphoma</u>

There are two types of cancer in one or more lymph nodes, Hodgkin's and non-Hodgkin's. The latter is by far the most common, often developing in people over 50, and may run in families. It may be triggered by a viral or bacterial infection, particularly after HIV/Aids when immunity is low. It is characterised by swelling in the groin, armpits, abdomen and neck, night sweats and loss of weight. Checks are needed to find out how far the disease has spread, which will require blood tests and scans. Treatment will be by radiotherapy or chemotherapy, with drugs to attach to and kill off cancer cells. Observation is needed after treatment to see that the cancer does not re-appear.

<u>Lung Cancer</u>

Lung cancer affects about 25,000 men each year in the UK, particularly those who have smoked for 20 or 30 years. It is possible for non-smokers to pick up cancer from regular contact with smokers and from pollution. Symptoms include coughing, wheezing, shortness of breath and chest pain. A tumour in the lungs may lead to pneumonia. Diagnosis will require X-rays, scans and possibly a bronchoscopy in which a flexible tube is passed into the lungs to take tissue samples. Treatment will probably require surgery, and either radiotherapy or chemotherapy.

Brain

Primary tumours in the brain can develop either on the neurons, or their tiny support system of glial cells, or in the cell membranes (meninges). Secondary tumours may have spread from other parts of the body. Symptoms include blurred vision, slurred speech, headaches, nausea, weakness and even seizure. A neurologist will probably call for X-rays and scans to see whether there are other tumours in the body. Treatment of primary tumours may involve drugs, radiotherapy, chemotherapy or even surgery, although this is often difficult to perform. Proton beam therapy or laser treatment under MRI control is likely to be safer. The prognosis for slow growing tumours in the meninges is quite good, but for aggressive tumours in the glial cells, the outlook is poor. Brain cancer affects about 11,000 people each year in the UK.

Stomach and Oesophagus

The incidence of stomach cancer is more common in older men, or those with blood group A and a family history. It usually starts in the stomach lining and spreads to other parts of the body. The causes are not properly understood, but gastritis and certain diets may increase the risks. Symptoms can include discomfort in the upper abdomen, stomach pains, loss of appetite and weight loss. Reporting symptoms early is important. Diagnosis will involve blood tests, ultrasound scans and X-rays after a barium meal. Treatment can require surgery or chemotherapy.

Bowel Cancer

Bowel, or colorectal cancer, is a tumour in the colon or rectum, occurring mainly in older men, and in a few cases is hereditary. Mostly, it occurs in the lower part of the colon and can be detected by a colonoscopy, a tube inserted into the rectum which can see polyps or tissue growth which may become cancerous. Symptoms include rectal discomfort, blood in the faeces, loss of appetite and even intestinal obstruction. Apart from a colonoscopy, diagnosis will involve blood tests, X-rays and scans. Treatment is likely to require immunotherapy drugs, radiotherapy and surgery, but chemotherapy will be needed if the cancer has metastasised. After surgery, a temporary or permanent colostomy may be required, in which faeces are passed out via a tube through the abdomen and into a bag. Early diagnosis is essential.

Immunotherapy

Understanding cancer and its treatment has advanced rapidly in recent years. One promising development is the use of immunotherapy drugs, which are applicable to most types of cancers. They inhibit the suppression of white blood cells, which are sent by the immune system to the sites of tumours to fight the cancer. As we have seen, cancer is usually caused by sustained damage to the DNA in our chromosomes and the subsequent failure of our immune system to recognise and destroy the cancer cells.

One of the main functions of white blood cells is to patrol the body, looking for infected and damaged cells. Cancer cells, which try to hide or are not very visible can only survive if they are not recognised by white blood cells and supressed. Inside a tumour, there are plenty of white blood cells, but they may not be effective in recognising and tackling cancer cells, and in some cases may even help the cancer cells. Immunotherapy drugs boost the immune system and encourage white blood cells to attack the cancers. It is now possible to remove white blood cells from a patient, modify them in a laboratory and reinsert them into the blood stream.

The latest drug called Ipilimumab, approved in 2011, is thought to be very promising, even in the last stages of metastasised cancers. It is a checkpoint inhibitor which unleashes the body's own T cells to fight the tumours. It is hoped that this and other immunotherapy drugs will drastically cut down mortality rates over the next 20 or 30 years.

Screening

It is clear that early diagnosis is vital for reducing mortality rates. Hence the importance of screening, which is now being trialled in certain UK cities, although there are risks of false readings and unwarranted interventions. Genetic kits are now available for assessing the risk of developing certain types of cancer, using samples of saliva, which should help early diagnosis.

CHAPTER 8

DEMENTIA AND ALZHEIMER'S

The Brain

As dementia and Alzheimer's are disorders of the brain, we should start off by looking at the workings of the brain. The brain is a very active part of the body, with a high metabolic demand. Dependant on nutrients from blood circulation, operating 24 hours a day, it uses up 15% of our glucose and 20% of our oxygen. It contains about 100 billion cells, or neurons, each attached to glial cells, connected to one another by synapses and messages are sent to one another by electrical signals, called neurotransmitters. There are seven different types of glia cells, each performing different functions. They protect and repair damaged neurons, assist the conductivity between neurons and fight infections and inflammation.

The brain is encased in a 3-layer membrane. The outer surface is multi-folded to be able to contain all the neurons. The brain is nourished by a cerebrospinal fluid (CSF), produced from ventricle cells, which removes toxins and waste particles, then is reabsorbed into the blood stream. Production of CSF decreases with age. There are two nervous systems emanating from the brain, the central nervous system, which runs down the spinal chord and the peripheral nervous system, which relays messages to all the organs and muscles in the body. The brain itself is composed of four distinct lobes. The temporal lobe deals with memory, hearing and emotion; the occipital lobe is responsible for vision; the parietal lobe processes sensory information; and the frontal lobe is responsible for decision making. Another key module inside the brain is the operational network, known as the basal ganglia which encases the two hippocampi, where memory is formed and retained.

Dementia

Dementia is a syndrome or disorder, starting with mild cognitive impairment, confusion and lack of reasoning ability, which usually gets progressively worse. About 70% of those who are affected go on to contract Alzheimer's disease. The cause of ordinary dementia might be depression, drugs, inflammation, tumours, sleeping problems and sudden change in personal circumstances, which are mostly treatable; but Alzheimer's is irreversible, even if it can be slowed down. There are well known cases of those who have been cured of Alzheimer's but almost certainly they had ordinary dementia and were wrongly diagnosed in the first place.

Alzheimer's

Alzheimer's disease generally affects older people and the incidence of Alzheimer's over the age of 65 is said to double every 5 years. Hence, the worldwide incidence of Alzheimer's rises as average lifespan increases. Women are more prone to the disease, possibly for hormonal reasons. The average duration of Alzheimer's is about 8 years from beginning to end. Patients do not usually die from the disease itself but from pneumonia. The symptoms include a decline in memory, speech, learning ability, recognising, understanding, reasoning, planning ability and motor skills. These are often accompanied by depression, stress, anxiety, loss of smell and poor sleep.

In the early stages a diagnosis for 'probable Alzheimer's' depends on scans and the number of symptoms. Although a number of biomarkers have been studied, there is no definitive test for most patients, other than at an autopsy, when a full examination of the brain is possible. But we do know the biological symptoms which are characterised by plaques and neurofibrillary tangles in the hippocampus and the cortex, the outer layer of cells in the brain. The plaques are small beta-amyloid proteins whilst the tangles between the neurons are phosphate tau proteins. Beta-amyloid proteins can actually be measured as Alzheimer's progresses, which is a useful diagnostic tool. However, plaques and tangles by themselves do not provide a perfect diagnosis, as they are also present in ordinary dementia patients, even from an early age.

As the disease progresses, the number of neurons in the brain diminishes, as it does to a lesser extent in normal ageing, and the brain shrinks in size. The neurons get damaged by DNA mutations, as do the body cells, which can lead to cancers, and communication between neurons via the synapses deteriorates. They can be repaired by glial cells or else commit apoptosis. Neurons cannot divide but can be replaced by neurogenesis in the hippocampus, whereby new cells are converted from stem cells. The hippocampus is generally the first module to be affected by Alzheimer's as short term memory deteriorates. This is followed up by loss of episodic memory, an inability to recall events, then historic memory and finally procedural memory, the ability to undertake tasks.

The next most common cause of dementia, after Alzheimer's, is vascular dementia, in which arteries conducting blood to the brain get blocked by a build up of plaques, as in atherosclerosis, which also leads to strokes. If the brain cannot get enough oxygen and nutrients from the blood, vascular dementia will deteriorate rapidly. Another disorder is called Lewy Body Disease, in which Lewy bodies, composed of a-synuclein, a special protein, damages the neurons, with similar symptoms to Alzheimer's and Parkinson diseases. Finally, Alzheimer's could be caused by a traumatic brain injury, either from a fall or from a contact sport.

Treatment

If Alzheimer's cannot be cured, can it be slowed down? There are a number of drugs which can slow it down and reduce depression, but only temporarily not permanently. Studies have shown that synaptic density limits the risk of Alzheimer's and slows its progress. This density is said to be increased by a number of factors, including education and learning, social activity, low blood pressure, adequate sleep, happiness, diet and exercise. Adequate sleep helps to clear up the toxins of the day. Happiness and well being is sometimes correlated with a high level of serotonin, derived from tryptophan, an amino acid, found in the digestive and central nervous systems. Diet includes adequate supplies of Vitamins B9 (folate), B12, C and and E, and trials have been undertaken to see if these really slow Alzheimer's down. In any event, a healthy diet, plenty of antioxidant foods, leafy vegetables, whole grains and oily fish, with high levels of Omega 3, are recommended. Marijuana, now approved for multiple sclerosis, may also be helpful in early stages of Alzheimer's.

Whilst treatment of Alzheimer's, sadly, is not effective in the long term, there are things we can do to help the patients, who are easy to irritate, can be aggressive, and also get very frustrated. Obviously we need to provide love and compassion, but we also need to try and make them feel valued. It is better not to contradict them and answer their questions patiently, even if they keep repeating them, and immediately forget the answer. As many patients cannot be allowed out alone, it is important to help them go for walks and get some exercise, give them a good diet, and keep them involved in some social activity, even if they can neither remember their friends nor make new ones.

Longer term, we can only hope that research will find better diagnostic tools, improved treatments and even a cure. The Alzheimer's Society has predicted that gene therapy injections may be helpful in the future. We shall see.

Chapter 9

WEIGHT, DIET AND FASTING

Our Metabolism

Before we look at weight issues and specific diets we should consider the factors which determine our shape and appearance. Clearly, most of this is due to our parents' genes and our lifestyle, but there are other factors involved.

The first is our metabolism, determined by our basal metabolic rate (BMR), that is to say the expenditure of energy over a given time, with the body at rest. About 70% of our energy is needed just to keep our blood circulation, breathing, digestion and muscle movement working. Those who have a high BMR will burn up calories and energy more quickly. So we see many people with a large appetite and a high BMR remaining slim, whilst those with a slow metabolism tending to put on weight. Our weight also depends on whether we have one or two FTO genetic risk factors, located on chromosome 16 and inherited from our parents, which predisposes us to put on weight. FTO genetic risk factors not only affect hunger and satiation, but are now being correlated with other medical disorders.

The incidence of obesity in the western world has increased steadily since the end of World War II, due to higher incomes, changes in taste, lower cost of food, more snack foods and sugary drinks, and possibly less exercise. In the USA for example, it is said that 60% of Americans are overweight or obese. In the UK we worry about the number of children who are overweight and what damage this might do to them in later life.

The BMI Index

One common measure of overweight is the BMI Index, which is calculated as your weight in kilograms, divided by your height in metres, squared. According to this index, for a person 5' 8" tall, his BMI would be as follows:

TABLE 1

Weight in		BMI
Stones	**Kilograms**	
9.25	60	18.5
11.5	72.5	25
13.8	88	30
18.5	117	35

A BMI regarded as normal is 18.5 to 25; a BMI 25 to 30 means overweight and over 30 is obese. A chart of the BMI Index is shown on page 60.

The Energy Fuels

So, let us look at how the whole metabolic process from eating to gaining weight takes place. There are two types of fuel for energy, glucose from carbohydrates, fatty acid from fatty food. When there is no carbohydrate available, the liver can convert protein into glucose.

In the digestive system, the body absorbs vitamins and minerals through the small intestine and colon. The food molecules are too large to be passed through the walls of the digestive tract and have to be broken down by digestive enzymes. Carbohydrates are broken down into glucose, fats into glycerol and fatty acid, and protein into amino acids. The tiny molecules can then be absorbed from the digestive tract into the blood stream.

Blood Sugar

The blood sugar, or glucose, in the blood stream gets transported into the body cells by a hormone transporter called insulin, where the ATP process, described earlier, turns it into energy for the muscles and organs. If we eat too much, and our energy needs are met, the liver turns the glucose into glycogen. When the glycogen storage facility is saturated, the liver converts glycogen into body fat for storage. When we eat too much, our blood sugar spikes and we need more insulin. Unfortunately, when we get fatter, the insulin receptors on our cell membranes get blocked, so our blood sugar and insulin levels remain high and the liver has no alternative but to convert the excess sugar into more fat.

Weight and Diabetes 2

As we saw in Chapter 6, when the cells start to block insulin and glucose, you can get Diabetes 2, as well as gaining extra weight. Diabetes may be due to genetic predisposition, but in the majority of cases, it is caused by diet. The incidence of Diabetes does increase with age, but can be prevented, or reversed if caught early, by cutting back on our food intake, changing the foods which we eat or stepping up our physical activity.

Carbohydrates

Over the years the percentage of carbohydrates to total macronutrients in our diet has increased. In the USA, for example, the percentage doubled between 1960 and 2000. Oddly enough, our total calorie intake has declined. The British Heart Foundation reported our average daily intake of calories fell from 2498 in 1975 to 2035 in 2010, whilst the daily fat intake fell from 112 grams to 84 grams. At the same time, obesity levels and Diabetes 2 have gone up. So what has gone wrong? Clearly the type of food, not the quantity, must be to blame. Whist our finger is often pointed at sugar, saturated fat, alcohol or too many snacks between meals, it is now being recognised that excess carbohydrate lies at the bottom of this puzzle. Alcohol, incidentally, whilst used as a fuel, cannot be stored in the liver like glucose, so it just substitutes for glucose, and it is the extra carbohydrates piled on top of alcohol which end up as fat.

Which Diets to Follow?

If we need to lose weight, which diets should we follow? I have looked at a number of diets, low calorie, low fat, low cholesterol, the Keswick diet, the Montignac diet, the Ketogenic diet, the Atkins diet, the 1:1 diet, the 5:2 diet, the Mayo clinic diet, the 'no breakfast' diet and the Glycemic Index diet, and will comment on those which are popular. However, whichever diet you follow there is a warning. When you diet your metabolism slows down and you burn up less calories!

Low Calorie Diet

The low calorie diet, probably the most popular, involves regular weight watching and studying calorie tables whist avoiding rich foods, alcohol and too much dining out. There is no question that reducing calories will reduce weight, but to take off 1 lb in weight, you have to forgo 3500 calories. A rapid weight reduction is obviously possible but this cannot easily be kept up for long, and a slow weight reduction over weeks or months gets very tedious. The chances are that when you stop your diet, the weight comes right back on. So that is why the low calorie diet is often nicknamed the yo-yo diet. To look at the amount of calories in each food, you can turn to the composition of 169 foods in Chapter 11.

Now, how many calories do we need each day? One calorie is the amount of energy required to heat one gram of water by one degree centigrade. An average male, aged 19-64, is recommended by Public Health England to consume 2500 calories per day, or 2342 for men over 65 and 2294 for men over 75, as we need less calories when we get older. As we raise our activity levels, the amount of calories we burn up rises sharply, as we can see from Table 2 below.

TABLE 2

Calorific Consumption per hour for selected activities	
Body at rest	70
Sitting	100
Eating	110
Driving	140
Housework	150
Cycling slowly	190
Walking briskly	290
Tennis, active	570
Swimming, distance	770
Road running	770
	Physiology of Exercise *Mulhouse and Miller*

What may be surprising is the amount of calories we need, even when we are asleep. To increase our daily calorie burn we obviously need to do some exercise like walking, but half an hour walking at normal pace does not use up a lot of calories. Suggestions for exercise are shown in Chapter 10.

The Ketogenic Diet

We now turn from the most popular to the least popular and most extreme diet, which some doctors neither like nor understand. The Ketogenic diet is sometimes associated with cancer management, but it can be used for other disorders, or just for weight loss. It was originally based on a modified metabolic theory that damage to the cells causing cancer starts with fermentation of glucose in the cytoplasm, the matter round the nucleus inside the cell membrane, not from accumulated DNA damage inside the nucleus. Cancer cells use 10 – 15 times more glucose to produce energy than normal cells, so the theory goes that one way to stop cancer cells proliferating is to starve them of glucose, rather than, as most oncologists advocate, to kill off cancer cells and boost the immune system. This has led to limited trials with humans, some using both methods to stop cancer spreading, particularly before and after chemotherapy. It has also been used successfully for epilepsy with children. However, we don't know how successful the Ketogenic diet, or a modified version, is going to be until more widespread trials have been undertaken. But at least it has led to better understanding of the role of carbohydrates and glucose, which is used in some of the diets which follow.

The Ketogenic diet itself is pretty drastic, cutting the percentage of carbohydrate in our diet from 45/65% to only 6% and cutting protein from 10/35% to 12%. This increases the fat content to 82%. The diet restricts the use of sugar, snacks, chocolates, processed food, fried food, alcohol, starchy vegetables, wheat, corn and specific oils for cooking. It encourages the use of high fat foods like butter, ghee, olive oil, coconut oil, nuts, oily fish and some meat. You are encouraged to eat plenty of leafy vegetables which are very low in protein and carbohydrate. It is possible to select the right foods for the diet, but very difficult to consume 2000 calories, or even 1000 calories a day as any meat or fish that you eat has a high protein content and you go over the limit of 12% of calories. Likewise it is difficult to consume 82% of 2000 calories (i.e. 1640 calories) in oils and fats, even if you use masses of olive oil in your salad dressing. So, it is recommended that you cut down your calories for only 5 days at a time. This means consuming 1100 calories on day one (500 for vegetables, 500 for nuts and oils and 100 for protein) and then on days 2 to 5 800 calories (400 for vegetables, 400 for nuts and oils). As part of the diet, you need to drink lots of water in order to keep down your LDL cholesterol and the risk of constipation.

Atkins and Other Low Carbohydrate Diets

Many diets like the Keswick, Montignac, Atkins and Mayo Clinic diets, also recommend low carbohydrates but allow far more protein, Atkins particularly. They also ban cakes, cookies, soft drinks, ice-cream and white bread, whilst warning about processed food using transfat or hydrogenated oil. The Atkins diet favours meat, fish, nuts, cheese, eggs, butter and leafy vegetables, avoiding starchy vegetables like potatoes which have a high carbohydrate content. If you cut out white flour, cereals and toast, you can transfer to coarse bran, flax seeds and nuts. Fibre is also recommended as it reduces blood sugar spikes, absorbs bacterial toxins, bulks up food in the intestines and avoids constipation. Fibre rich foods include most vegetables, nuts, seeds, beans, legumes, fruit and unrefined grains. Both the UK and US Health Authorities recommend a minimum of 30 grams of fibre per day, and say that modern diets are inadequate.

The Glycemic Index Diet

Many foods recommended by Atkins are low glycemic, which is classed as a diet on its own. The Glycemic Index or GI Index, ranging from 0 to 100, shows the percentage sugar in the food, sugar or glucose reading 100. You may also have heard of a similar index called Glycemic Load. This takes account of the average portion size of any food you eat, multiplied by the GI Index and divided by 100. Most breads, pastries and cereals, apart from All Bran, are high glycemic, as is white rice. Fruits are mostly below 50, as are legumes. Particularly low are lentils, 29, Kidney beans, 27, and peanuts, only 14. Starchy vegetables are usually high, like baked potato, 85. In the tables on the Composition of Foods, Chapter 11, you will see a special column showing the glycemic index of all 169 foods.

The Mayo Clinic Diet

This is a two-week diet. Day 1 starts off with half a grapefruit, 3 eggs and black coffee for breakfast, 3 eggs and coffee for lunch, and half a grapefruit, 3 eggs and salad for dinner. In each of the following days, eat grapefruit, 3 or 4 eggs, spinach, salad, fish, meat or chicken, and, of course, black coffee. The Clinic claims that the eggs set up a chemical reaction and that 15-20 lbs can be lost in 2 weeks. Obviously no carbohydrate here, but watch out for looking a bit yellow!

The 'No Breakfast' and the 16-hour diet

A typical Mediterranean diet includes fish, meat, fruit, vegetables and wine, with minimal carbohydrates for breakfast, possibly only a croissant and coffee. The 'no breakfast' diet goes one step further, no croissant!

It is known that blood sugar spikes after a meal, and spikes higher after the first meal of the day than after subsequent meals. The normal blood sugar level for healthy people who eat three meals a day is about 5 mmol/L, rising to 8 mmol/L after a meal. In a study of diabetics, the blood sugar level rose from 8 mmol/L to 10 mmol/L after breakfast, but averaged only 7 mmol/L all day, if they omitted breakfast.

The main reason was avoiding processed cereals at breakfast which are highly glycemic.

The advantage of a 'no breakfast' diet is not just that it cuts out some carbohydrates and calories but it allows a period of 16 hours between the end of dinner the night before and lunch next day. During this fasting period the body will use up glucose from the last meal and possibly reduce the store of glycogen in the liver, which might otherwise be turned into fat. I believe it is time to disregard the old fashioned advice, promoted by cereal manufacturers and supported by some doctors, that we should "eat breakfast like a king, lunch like a prince and dine like a pauper."

The 5:2 and 1:1 Diets

A recently popular diet is the 5:2 diet, a form of intermittent fasting. It is claimed that this is less boring and easier to manage than dieting every day. For two days out of five, or one day out of two in the 1:1 diet, calories are restricted to 600 per day, whilst eating freely on the other days. During these periods of fasting, as with the 16-hour diet above, glycogen can be released from the liver for energy.

Supplements

It is said that you don't need any supplements if you have a balanced diet, except perhaps Vitamin D for older people in the winter. But when you are fasting, or on a diet, your diet is certainly not balanced. You could take a multivitamin with Vitamins ABCDE of which Vitamin B is probably the most important. One mineral you could need is Magnesium which plays a role in over three hundred biochemical reactions in the body and has an important role in the production of ATP. Three other supplements are sometimes suggested – Co-enzyme Q10 (CoQ10), L-carnitine and PQQ, (Pyrroloquinoline Quinone).

CoQ10 is a soluble vitamin-like molecule, produced in our cells, but production declines with age. Various medications like statins are said to deplete CoQ10 so it could be useful as a supplement. CoQ10 is a membrane stabilizer, an antioxidant, and it plays a key role in the Electronic Chain, referred to in Chapter 1. It is present in nearly all cells and is essential to life. As an antioxidant, it can prevent the oxidation of LDL cholesterol and lowers blood pressure. Supplements are available for 100-300 mg per day, some in the form of ubiquinol.

L-carnitine is similar to CoQ10 and acts as transporter of fatty acids through the membranes of the mitochondria where ATP is produced, and also clears the build up of lactic acid during strenuous physical activity. Three quarters of L-carnitine that we need comes from dietary intake, including red meat, poultry, fish and dairy products, but a quarter is synthesised within our bodies. However, body synthesis, as with CoQ10, declines with age. L-carnitine could be more useful if you are on a high fat diet as it is the only fat transporter used for energy. Supplements are available for 1 gram per day.

PQQ is a soluble vitamin, possibly a previously unidentified B vitamin, protecting the nerve cells, stimulating the growth of mitochondria and protecting them from oxidative damage. It is possible, but not yet proven that boosting the number of mitochondria in each cell may lead to increased longevity. PQQ can be found in certain fruits and vegetables, human breast milk, legumes, cocoa powder and chocolate. Supplements are available for 20 mg per day.

Perhaps we should also mention probiotic supplements which increase the concentration of friendly bacteria in our gut and help our digestive system. However, probiotic foods like live cultured yoghurt, fibre rich foods, fermented foods like sauerkraut or anti-oxidant fruit and vegetables mentioned in Table 5 will do just as well.

<u>Diet Conclusions</u>

There are, I believe, a number of lessons we can learn from all these diets. I have listed ten.

1. Excess carbohydrate should be avoided.
2. Saturated fats are not bad for you if you eat a balanced diet.
3. Straight forward calorie counting and weight watching are very boring on a permanent basis, and intermittent calorie restrictions may end up as yo-yo dieting.
4. The Ketogenic diet seems too extreme, except for just a 5-day trial, but it is effective in the short term.
5. The 16-hour daily fast is easier than the 5:2 or 1:1 diets.
6. A modest calorie reduction of 200-300 calories a day is safer and more manageable than a drastic reduction in calories.
7. Some supplements might be advisable if our normal dietary pattern is changed during a strict diet.
8. Various foods like oily fish, legumes, fermented foods, leafy vegetables and even dark chocolate are recommended, whilst processed food and hydrogenated oils are definitely out.
9. Try to stick to low glycemic foods.
10. An increase in physical activity burns up more calories, as we shall see in the next chapter.

<u>Which foods to eat?</u>

There is a bewildering mass of articles and advice from nutritionists, biochemists and doctors on which foods we should eat, and which to avoid, to keep us healthy. The former include dark chocolate, red wine, turmeric, green tea, fermented foods, rye bread, coffee, nuts, rich cheese, oily fish and all the fruit and vegetables which are anti-oxidant, shown in Table 5. So it is hard to give advice. I suggest, just use your common sense and enjoy!

TABLE 3

Body Mass Index Chart

Index	19	20	21	22	23	24	25	26	27	28	29	30	31	32	33	34	35
Height (feet/ inches)								*Body Weight (pounds)*									
4'10"	91	96	100	105	110	115	119	124	129	134	138	143	148	153	158	162	167
4'11"	94	99	104	109	114	119	124	128	133	138	143	148	153	158	163	168	173
5'	97	102	107	112	118	123	128	133	138	143	148	153	158	163	168	174	179
5'1"	100	106	111	116	122	127	132	137	143	148	153	158	164	169	174	180	185
5'2"	104	109	115	120	126	131	136	142	147	153	158	164	169	175	180	186	191
5'3"	107	113	118	124	130	135	141	146	152	158	163	169	175	180	186	191	197
5'4"	110	116	122	128	134	140	145	151	157	163	169	174	180	186	192	197	204
5'5"	114	120	126	132	138	144	150	156	162	168	174	180	186	192	198	204	210
5'6"	118	124	130	136	142	148	155	161	167	173	179	186	192	198	204	210	216
5'7"	121	127	134	140	146	153	159	166	172	178	185	191	196	204	211	217	223
5'8"	125	131	138	144	151	158	164	171	177	184	190	197	203	210	216	223	230

5'9"	128	135	142	149	155	162	169	176	182	189	196	203	209	216	223	230	236
5'10"	132	139	146	153	160	167	174	181	188	195	202	209	216	222	229	236	243
5'11"	136	143	150	157	165	172	179	186	193	200	208	215	222	229	236	243	250
6'	140	147	154	162	169	177	184	191	199	206	213	221	228	235	242	250	258
6'1"	144	151	159	166	174	182	189	197	204	212	219	227	235	242	250	257	265
6'2"	148	155	163	171	179	186	194	202	210	218	225	233	241	249	256	264	272
6'3"	152	160	168	176	184	192	200	208	216	224	232	240	248	256	264	272	279
6'4"	156	164	172	180	189	197	205	213	221	230	238	246	254	263	271	279	287

Source: Clinical Guidelines on the Identification, Evaluation, and Treatment of Overweight and Obesity in Adults, US National Institute of Health, National Heart, Lung, and Blood Institute, June 1998.

CHAPTER 10

EXERCISE

As we saw earlier, we burn up calories even when we are sleeping or not doing anything. However, the body needs some activity to keep our muscles working, particularly our heart muscles and respiratory system. Bones can actually strengthen if you do some exercise, or they can lose mass if you are inactive, as astronauts can testify. Walking helps, at least 30 minutes a day, but sustained walking at a brisk pace is far better. For older men, the thought of brisk walking or specific exercises is rather daunting. It is certainly easier to walk at a measured pace, not forcing ourselves to stride out and increase the pace. But it does get easier once you begin and becomes part of your daily routine.

For those on a diet, you have to burn up a lot of calories, 3500, to lose just one pound of weight. This could mean putting in an extra 350 calories of energy per day for 10 days. But exercise should not be regarded as being needed only for those on a diet. It has other effects, such as providing a sense of well being, which is now thought to be due to an increase in serotonin, or, as athletes put it, to 'runners high'.

If you are now retired, gardening, walking, cycling, golf, tennis, jogging, dancing, sailing, riding, skiing, or swimming, any of these should help to keep you active. Walking an hour a day should be sufficient if you can increase the pace for 20 minutes. Ideally, whatever your exercise, you should raise your heart rate for at least 12 minutes a day, from say 70 to over 100 and the latest 'fitbit' watch will be able to tell tell you that. If you want to speed up walking, try using hiking sticks which also exercises the upper body. It is also helpful to undertake some form of stress exercise where there is resistance to your arm or leg movements, like pulling, pushing and lifting, which build up the muscles.

Callisthenics, bending, stretching and lifting may look rather undignified, but you could take part in an exercise class, or do Pilates, T'ai Chi or Yoga in a group. Alternatively, if you have a static bicycle machine, a rowing machine, or a running board, you can do all this in your own home. One of the best regimes, designed by the Royal Canadian Air Force in the late 50's is the 5Bx programme, available in print or on the internet. This asks you to do five exercises, allowing a number of minutes for each exercise, graded according to difficulty. The exercises comprise stretching, sit-ups, back extension, push-ups and running in place.

Exercise does not only improve your posture and your metabolism, it improves your appetite and leaves you in a better mood. In the cells themselves, it may increase the number of mitochondria, give the cells more capacity to produce energy and help to balance the level of free radicals in your cells, which could otherwise lead to oxidation. Very strenuous exercise should be avoided for older men, which could cause free radical damage, but, overall, a reasonable degree of exercise should lower the health risks for older men. I am told the Harvard Rowing Eight of 1912, rowed together over the Henley course in 1964, all in their mid-70's. That is probably a tall ask for most of us, but taking the effort to do something regularly, avoid being inactive, walking not driving, taking the stairs not the lift, carrying the shopping and even lifting the grandchildren, will all help. If it burns up unwanted calories, so much the better. Otherwise, follow the diet recommendations on page 73.

CHAPTER 11

THE COMPOSITION OF FOODS

The tables showing the composition of 169 foods on pages 43-49 are quite detailed, so before looking at the numbers or symbols, I suggest that you first look through the meaning of each of the headings, starting with calories.

Calories

The calorie levels in column 1 are shown for 100 grams of food or 100 m/l drink. These figures, and also those in columns 6-8 are taken from the acclaimed 'Composition of Foods' 7th edition, by McCance and Widdowson, used by most nutritionists.

The daily calorie allowance recommended by Public Health England for men over 65 is 2342 and 2294 for those over 75, but would be more for those doing heavy work or being much more active.

GI Values

The second column shows the GI (Glycemic Index) values for each food, as described on page 68 in Chapter 9. The index shows the percentage of sugar in each food from 0 to 100. Where there is no sugar, or only a negligible amount, it is shown as 'n'. For anyone following a GI diet, the aim is to avoid foods with a rating over 50, or at least over 55. For breakfast eaters, this probably means a change in their choice of foods.

Macronutrients

Columns 3-5 show the percentage of macronutrients, that is protein, fat and carbohydrate in each food.

Proteins

Proteins are not principally used for energy although they can be used if fat or carbohydrate is not available. Protein is mainly needed for growth and body renewal. The main protein content in our food is provided by meat, fish, eggs and cheese.

Carbohydrates

This is our main source of energy and quickest to digest: Carbohydrates take the form of single, double and multisugars (polysaccharides) together with cellulose. The single sugars, glucose and fructose, found in fruit and vegetables, are digested the quickest. Double sugars are found in sucrose (sugar), lactose (milk) and maltose (beer) whilst multisugars are mainly found in grains, cereals, bread and potatoes.

Fats

The richest source of energy are fats. They provide more than twice the amount of energy (weight for weight) produced by carbohydrate, but we eat much less of it. Chemically, fat contains three fatty acids, saturated, monounsaturated, polyunsaturated and also transfat. Saturated fat is commonly found in meat, butter, cheese, whole milk and ice cream. Monounsaturated fat is found in nuts, oils and red meat. Polyunsaturated fat is split into Omega 3 and Omega 6 fatty acids, neither of which can be synthesised in our bodies, and we need small amounts in our diet. Omega 3 has two forms, 'short chain' found in flaxseed, walnuts and rapeseed oil. 'Long chain' is found in oily fish, such as salmon, mackerel, sardines, herring, trout and shellfish. Our main source of transfat is from industrially produced margarine, cooking fats and other processed foods. Transfat has been shown to raise cholesterol levels and is now gradually being phased out.

<u>Micronutrients</u>

Columns 6 and 7 show the percentage of vitamins and minerals in each food. These are needed generally in tiny quantities, sometimes as little as millionths of a gram. I have selected only the key vitamins and minerals which we need and these are shown in the tables in a chemical letter format (to save space) alongside the quantity recommended for consumption each day, for males aged up to 64, according to Public Health England.

TABLE 4

Vitamins		Chemical Letter Format	Recommended daily allowance mg or mcg[1]
A		A	700 mcg
B1	Thiamin	t	1 mg
B2	Riboflavin	r	1.3 mg
B3	Niacin	n	16.5 mg
B6	Pyridoxine	B6	1.4 mg

---

[1] 1 mg is one thousandth of a gram. 1 mcg is one millionth of a gram.

B12	Cobalamin	B12	1.5 mcg
B	Folate	f	200 mcg
C		C	40 mg
D		D	10 mcg
E		E	15 mg *
Minerals			
Potassium		K	4.7 mg *
Calcium		Ca	800 mg
Magnesium		Ma	350 mg
Phosphorous		P	550 mg
Iron		Fe	6 mg
Sodium Chloride		SCL	2.5 grams *

In the tables, columns 6 and 7, vitamins and minerals, are ONLY shown if they provide at least ONE THIRD of the UK daily recommended allowance. What surprised me in preparing the tables was how so few foods provided more than two or three vitamins and minerals which contained over one third of our daily allowance per 100 grams. One of the reasons is that we may eat more than 100 grams (3½ ounces) of any one food at a sitting. The second reason is they all add up. Even if one food has a tiny amount and another has a tiny amount, they all add up and hopefully keep us healthy.

Before we move on to column 8, fibre, I will summarise what each of these vitamins and minerals does:

---

* UK Health Authorities do not give a recommended daily allowance. This is the USA recommendation.

<u>Vitamins</u>

Vitamin A   Helps to maintain body tissue. Composed of retinol, found in liver, oily fish and dairy products; and also carotene, found in carrots, red peppers, sprouts and other vegetables.

Thiamin   Helps convert carbohydrates into energy. Found in whole grains, meat, milk, cheese, eggs and vegetables. Removed from flour in milling and added back to certain foods.

Riboflavin   Also used for energy conversion. Found in milk, liver and kidneys. Added back to white bread and cereals.

Niacin   Also used for energy conversion. Added to white flour and cereals. Rich sources are meat, poultry, liver and fish.

Pyridoxine   Involved in metabolism of amino acids. Widely found in whole grains, meat, liver, chicken, fish and eggs. Sometimes added to cereals.

Cobalamin   Needed for cell division, blood formation and neurological function. Sources include organic meats, fish and dairy products. Sometimes added to cereals.

Folate Needed for cell division. Low levels in a wide variety of foods. Added to cereals.

Vitamin C Needed for energy conversion, blood circulation and formation of tissue. Can not be synthesised in the body and therefore needed in the diet. It is an important antioxidant. Found mainly in fruit and vegetables, but can easily be destroyed by cooking.

Vitamin D Responsible for bone formation and absorption of minerals. Mainly obtained from ultra violet rays absorbed through the skin.

Vitamin E A fat soluble anti-oxidant which helps maintain our cell structure and muscle tissue. Sources include whole grains, vegetable oils, fatty meat, vegetables and yeast.

Vitamin K Needed for clotting of blood. Main sources are pulses and leafy vegetables.

Minerals

Calcium 99% found in bones and teeth. Needed also for muscle contraction. Found in milk, cheese, nuts, beans and vegetables.

Magnesium Needed for muscles and energy conversion. Found in whole grains, nuts, spices and leafy vegetables.

Potassium   Found in inter cellular fluids, works with sodium for cell functioning. Found in fruit, vegetables and many other foods.

Sodium Chloride   Present in blood and body fluids, helps to maintain our electrolyte balance. Sources are processed and preserved food, used in cooking or added to our food. We need about 2-3 grams a day but often consume too much.

Iron   Needed for red blood cells. Helps transfer oxygen from our lungs to our tissues. Available in meat, poultry, fish, pulses and whole grains.

Fibre Column 8 shows the percentage fibre content in each food. Mostly provided by cereals, nuts, pulses, fruit and vegetables. We need 30 grams per day which many western diets don't provide. Fibre is important for our gut bacteria. Affects our whole digestive process and our health in general.

Acid and Alkali Column 9 shows whether the food is acid or alkali forming. Acid is marked 'c', Alkaline is marked 'k'. The balance between acid and alkaline contents in our cells and body fluid is measured on a scale called 'potential hydrogen' or PH, which can range from 0 to 14. Human blood stays between a narrow range from 7.35 and 7.45, and any deviation can be dangerous. If we consume too much acid forming food and drink, the enzyme activity in our metabolism which controls our digestion is adversely affected. The PH level falls, the nutrients are less easily absorbed and we may get indigestion. Most foods are acid forming, but fruit and vegetables, which are alkaline, come to the rescue.

Anti-oxidants In column 10, foods which are anti-oxidant are marked 'a-ox'. Anti-oxidants are produced both in our bodies and in the foods we eat, most fruit and vegetables. Anti-oxidants are important for neutralising the free radicals in our cells.

TABLE 5

The Composition of Foods

FOOD	Calories per 100 gms/ml	GI Values n=negligible	% composition of each food		
			Protein	Fat	Carbohydrate
CEREALS					
Rice, white, Basmati	351	58	8	1	84
Rice, brown, raw	333	70	8	2	77
Wholewheat pasta, spaghetti	329	42	13	3	68
Bread, white	230	70	8	2	47
Bread, thick wholemeal	217	73	9	3	42
Bran cereal, fortified	267	74	12	3	50
Cornflakes, fortified	376	77	7	1	91
Muesli	366	56	9	6	73
Porridge oats, unfortified	381	42	11	8	71
Rice Krispies, fortified	374	82	6	1	91
Shredded Wheat, unfortified	333	75	11	3	71
Weetabix, unfortified	332	74	11	2	73
Cream crackers	445	65	9	16	70
Fruit cake, homemade	334	54	5	12	55
Sponge cake	463	46	6	25	53
Pastry, flaky, uncooked	384	59	5	26	34
Doughnuts	321	76	5	13	48
DAIRY PRODUCTS					
Semi-skimmed milk	46	20	4	2	5
Whole milk	63	31	3	4	5
Condensed milk, sweetened	310	61	7	8	56
Soya milk, fortified, sweetened	43	36	3	2	3
Camembert cheese	290	n	21	22	
Cheddar cheese	416	n	25	35	
Cottage cheese, plain	103	n	9	6	3
Stilton cheese	410	n	23	35	
Goat's cheese	320	n	21	26	1
Yoghurt, Greek style, fruit	137	31	4	1	13
Ice cream, soft scoop, vanilla	169	61	3	8	22
Chocolate ice cream	295	37	3	22	23
EGGS					
Chicken eggs	131	n	13	9	
FATS		n			
Butter	744	n	1	82	1
Margarine	688	n		76	
Dripping, beef	891	n		99	
Cod liver oil	899	n		100	
Olive oil	899	n		100	

Nutrients over 33% of required intake		% Fibre in gms	Acid (c) or Alkaline (k)	a-ox if anti-oxidant
Vitamins	Minerals			
		1.1	c	
	Mg P	3.0	c	
t n	Mg P Fe	11.7	c	
		2.8	c	
	P	7.0	c	
D t r n 6 12 f	Ca Mg Fe	24.6	c	
D t r n 6 12		2.6	c	
n 6	P	8.8	c	
t	Mg P Fe	7.8	c	
D t r n 6 12 f	P Fe	0.7	c	
	P	12.2	c	
n	Mg P Fe	9.7	c	
		3.9	c	
		1.3	c	
A 12	P	1.1	c	
		2.8	c	
		1.7	c	
12			c	
12			c	a-ox
r 12	Ca P		c	
		0.5	c	a-ox
A r 12 f	Ca P Cl		c	
A 12	Ca P Cl		c	
12			c	
A r 12 f	Ca P Cl		c	
12	Cl		c	
			c	
		0.2	c	
			c	
r 12			c	
A	Cl		c	
A D E	Cl		c	
			c	
A D E			k	a-ox
E			k	a-ox

Sunflower oil	899	n		100	
MEAT AND POULTRY					
Bacon rashers, back	215	n	17	17	
Ham	107	n	18	3	1
Gammon steak	138	n	18	8	
Beef, lean, raw	129	n	23	4	
Minced beef	225	n	18	16	
Veal escalope, fried	196	n	33	7	
Lamb, lean, raw	153	n	20	8	
Lamb chops, lean and fat	277	n	18	23	
Pork, lean, raw	123	n	22	4	
Pork chops, lean and fat	270	n	19	22	
Chicken meat, average, raw	108	n	22	2	
Turkey meat, average, raw	105	n	23	2	
Duck meat, raw	137	n	20	7	
Venison	165	n	36	2	
Kidney, lamb	188	n	24	10	
Liver, calf	176	n	22	10	
Corned beef	205	n	26	11	1
Liver pâté	349	n	13	33	1
Pork sausages, raw	309	28	12	25	10
FISH					
Cod, raw	75	n	18	1	
Haddock, raw	75	n	18		
Plaice, raw	76	n	17	1	
Anchovies, canned in oil, drained	191	n	25	10	
Kippers, grilled	245	n	22	18	
Mackerel, raw	233	n	18	18	
Salmon, raw	217	n	20	15	
Smoked salmon	184	n	23	10	
Sardines, canned in oil, drained	220	n	23	14	
Tuna, canned, in oil drained	159	n	25	6	
Prawns, King, raw	77	n	18	1	
Mussels, cooked, no shells	104	n	18	2	3
Fish fingers, grilled	223	n	14	9	22
Fish paste	170	n	15	11	4
VEGETABLES					
New potatoes, boiled in skin	64	76	2		15
Old potatoes, peeled	82	76	2		20
Chips, oven ready, baked	189	57	3	5	35
Potato crisps	493	74	6	29	56
Baked beans	81	48	5	1	15
Beans, green, raw	24	n	2		3
Broad beans	48	63	5	1	6
Butter beans, canned	77	36	6	1	13
Chick peas, boiled	121	5	8	2	18

E			c	a-ox
t n 6	Cl		c	
t n 6	P Cl	0.1*	c	
t	Cl		c	
6 12	P		c	
n 12			c	
n 6 12	P		c	
12			c	
12			c	
t n 6 12	P		c	
t 6 12			c	
n			c	
n 6 12	P		c	
t r n 12	P		c	
r n 6 12	P Fe		c	
t r n 6 12 f	P Fe		c	
A t r n 6 12 f	P Fe		c	
12	Cl		c	
A r 12 f	Cl Fe	0.6	c	
12		2.8	c	
12			c	
12			c	
t 12			c	
12	Ca P Fe Cl		c	
D 12	P Cl		c	
D n 12	P		c	
D t n 12	P	0.2	c	a-ox
D t n 6 12	P Cl		c	a-ox
D n 12	Ca P		c	
n 12	P		c	
12			c	a-ox
12	p Fe		c	a-ox
	12	2.0	c	
	Ca P	2.6	c	
		1.8	k	
C		2.0	c	
		3.8	k	
E	K Cl			
t f		4.9	c	
		3.4	k	
		4.6*		
		4.6*	c	
f	P Cl	4.3*		

Lentils, raw	318	30	24	1	54
Kidney beans, raw	266	36	22	1	44
Runner beans, raw	22	n	2		3
Peas, raw	83	39	7	2	11
Asparagus	25	n	2	1	2
Broccoli, raw	34	n	4	1	3
Brussels sprouts, raw	42	n	3	1	4
Cabbage, raw	27	n	2		4
Carrots, young, raw	30	49	1		6
Cauliflower, raw	30	n	2		4
Celery, raw	7	n	1		1
Courgette, raw	18	n	2		2
Cucumber	14	n	1	1	1
Curley kale, raw	33	n	3	2	1
Garlic	98	n	8	1	16
Leeks, raw	22	n	2	1	3
Lettuce, raw	11	n	1		2
Mushrooms, raw	7	n	1		
Onions, raw	35	n	1		8
Parsnip, raw	64	91	2	1	12
Red Peppers. Raw	21	n			4
Sauerkraut, bottled, drained	9	n	1		1
Spinach, raw	25	n	0	3	1
Sweetcorn, boiled	34	48	3		3
Tomatoes, raw	14	n	1		3
Watercress, raw	22	n	3	1	
HERBS AND SPICES					
Basil, fresh	40	n	3	1	5
Chilli powder	n	n	13	14	
Coriander leaves	18	n	12	18	
Cumin Seeds	n	n	18	22	
Ginger, fresh	44	n	2	1	8
Paprika	n	n	14	13	
Parsley, fresh	34	n	3	1	3
Pepper, black	n	n	10	3	
Rosemary, dried	331	n	5	15	48
Thyme, dried	276	n	9	7	45
FRUIT					
Apples, eating	51	38	1	1	12
Apricots, raw	51	57	1		7
Avocado	31	n	2	20	2
Bananas, flesh only	81	52	1		20
Blackberries, raw	25	40	1		5
Blueberries	40	53	1		9
Cherries	48	22	1		12
Dates (stoned)	270	103	3		68

t 6	P Fe	4.9*	k	
t f	K Mg P Fe	15.7*	c	a-ox
C		2.0*	k	
A C t		5.3	k	a-ox
A f		1.7*	k	a-ox
A C f		2.5*	k	a-ox
C f		4.1*	k	a-ox
A C t		4.1	k	a-ox
A		3.9	k	a-ox
C		1.8	k	a-ox
		1.1*	k	a-ox
A C		0.9*	k	a-ox
		0.7	k	
C f			k	a-ox
C		4.1*	k	a-ox
6 C		2.2*	k	a-ox
		1.5	k	a-ox
		0.7	k	
		2.2	k	a-ox
C f		4.7	k	
A C f		2.2		a-ox
	Cl	2.2*	c	
A C f		2.1*	c	a-ox
C		2.0*	k	
A C		1.0	c	a-ox
A C		1.5*	k	
A C	Ca			a-ox
A r n 6	K Ca Mg P Fe Cl	34.8		a-ox
C n	K Ca Mg P Fe	41.9	k	a-ox
A t	K Ca Mg P Fe	10.5		a-ox
		2.0	k	a-ox
A t r n 6	K CA Mg P Fe	34.9		a-ox
A C f	Fe		k	a-ox
A	K Ca Mg Fe	25.3		a-ox
A C t r 6 f	Ca Mg Fe	42.6		a-ox
A C t 6 f	Ca Mg P Fe	37.0		a-ox
		1.2	k	a-ox
A		1.7*	k	a-ox
		3.4*	k	
		1.4	k	
E C		3.1*	k	a-ox
		1.5	c	a-ox
C			k	a-ox
		4.0*	c	a-ox

Figs	209	61	3	2	49
Grapefruit, flesh only	30	30	1		7
Grapes, green, seedless	62	53	1		15
Lemons, whole, no pips	19	42	1		3
Melon, flesh only Canteloupe	19	47	1		4
Olives, green	103	n	1		11
Oranges, flesh only	30	42	1		8
Peaches, flesh and skin	33	42	1		8
Pears, flesh and skin	43	38			11
Pineapple, flesh only	41	66			10
Plums, flesh and skin	36	24	1		9
Prunes, semi dried	141	29	3		34
Raisins	272	64	2		69
Rhubarb, stewed	48	n	1		11
Strawberries	30	40	1	1	6
SOUPS AND SAUCES					
Chicken soup, canned	58	50	1	4	5
Mushroom soup, canned	46	50	1	3	4
Tomato soup, canned	51	38	9	2	8
Vegetable soup, canned	39	39	1	1	7
French dressing	335	n		32	12
Mayonnaise	686	n	1	75	2
Mint sauce	101	n	1		21
Soy sauce	79	n	3		18
Salt, table	n	n			
Vinegar	22	n			1
SUGAR AND PRESERVES					
Honey	288	55			76
Jam, fruit	261	56	1		69
Marmalade	261	48			70
Sugar, white	394	65			100
Chocolate, plain	510	20	5	28	64
Mars bar	404	62	4	15	66
Liquorice Allsorts	349	78	3	5	77
NUTS AND SEEDS					
Almonds	612	24	21	56	7
Brazil nuts	683	24	15	68	3
Peanuts, plain	564	14	15	26	37
Walnuts	688	n	15	68	3
Sesame seeds	598	n	18	53	1
Sunflower seeds	576	n	20	48	19
BEVERAGES					
Cocoa, powder	312	n	19	22	12
Coffee, instant powder	75	n	15		5
Tea, black, infused	0	n			
Tea, green, infused	0	n			

	Fe	6.9*	c	a-ox
C		1.3*	k	a-ox
		1.2	k	
C			k	a-ox
A C		1.8	k	a-ox
	Cl	2.9*	k	a-ox
C		1.2	k	a-ox
C		1.5*	k	a-ox
		2.7	k	a-ox
		1.2*	k	
A		1.6*	K	a-ox
		2.4*	c	a-ox
	Fe	2.0*	k	a-ox
		1.2*	c	
C		1.0*	k	a-ox
			c	
		0.1*	c	
A		0.6	c	
		1.5*		
		0.5*	c	
E			c	
	Fe		c	
r n	Cl		k	a-ox
	Cl		c	
			c	
			k	
			c	
		0.5	c	
			c	
		2.5*	c	
		0.8	c	
	Fe	2.0*		a-ox
E r	Ca Mg P Fe	7.4*	k	a-ox
E t	Mg P	4.3*	c	a-ox
E t n 6 f	Mg P	6.2*	c	a-ox
t 6 f	Mg P Fe	7.5*	c	a-ox
t 6 f	Ca Mg P Fe	7.9*	k	a-ox
E t	Mg P Fe	6.0*	k	a-ox
	Fe	12.1*	c	a-ox
n	K Mg P Fe		c	
			c	a-ox
			k	a-ox

Coke Cola	41	53			11
Lemonade	22	54			6
Tonic water	22	53			6
Orange juice	36	53	1		9
Tomato juice	14	8	1		3

			c	
			c	
			c	
C		0.2*	c	a-ox
		0.6*	c	a-ox

REFERENCES AND SOURCES

The Composition of Foods, 7th edition, *McCance and Widdowson*

The Association of UK Dieticians

Principles of Anatomy and Physiology, *Tortora and Grabowski*

BMA Complete Home Medical Guide

Molecular Biology of Cancer, *Lauren Pecorino*

Targeted Cancer Treatments, *Elaine Vickers*

Mitochondria and the Future of Medicine, *Lee Know*

Osteoarthritis, *Prieto-Alhambra, Arden and Hunter*

The Cerebro Standstill, *Meenakshi Narang*

Stroke, *Richard I Lindley*

Osteoporosis, *Black, Sandison and Reid*

Tumours and Cancers, *Dongyou Liu*

Put your Heart in your Mouth, *Dr. Campbell McBride*

The Longevity Diet, *Dr. Valter Longo*

Keto for Cancer, *Miriam Kalamian*

Alzheimer's Disease Decoded, *Sahyouni, Verma and Chen*

Cancer and its Management, *Tobias and Hochhauser*

Prostate Cancer, *Mason and Moffat*

The Telomere Effect, *Blackburn and Elissa Epel*

Breakfast is a Dangerous Meal, *Terence Kealy*

Alzheimer's Disease and Dementia, *Steven Sabat*

Diabetes, *Matthews, Beatty, Dyson, King, Meston, Pal and Shaw*

Heart Disease, *Lynne McTaggart*

New Diet Revolution, *Dr. Atkins*

Google Scholar and Wikipedia

The Shoppers Guide to GI Values, *Brand-Miller, Foster-Powell and Atkinson*

The Glycemic Load Counter, *Mable Blades*

ABOUT THE AUTHOR

In his late eighties, Shaun Dowling, former marathon runner and still rowing on the Thames, looks at how the body works and what can go wrong for older men. In his book he covers eight possible medical disorders, prostate, heart, strokes, osteoarthritis, osteoporosis, diabetes, cancer and dementia, how to spot them, how to treat them, and, where possible, how to avoid them in the first place. He then goes on to discuss weight problems, diet and exercise.